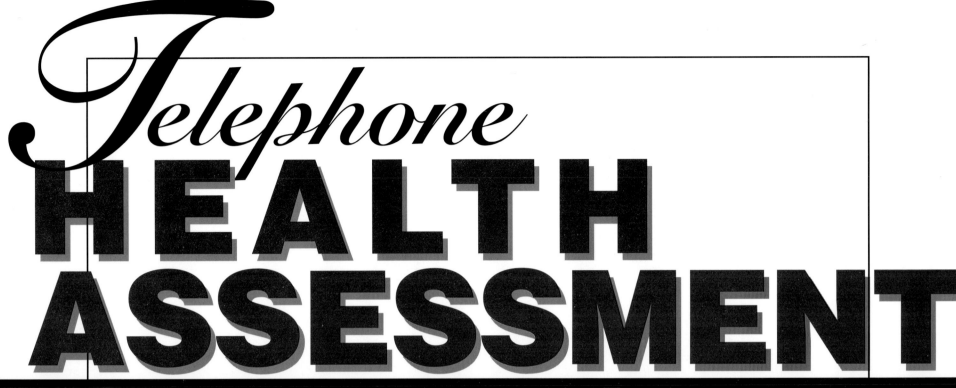

Telephone HEALTH ASSESSMENT
GUIDELINES FOR PRACTICE

Sandra M. Simonsen, RN, MSN
Kaiser Permanente, Anaheim, California

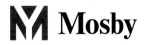

Mosby

St. Louis Baltimore Boston Carlsbad Chicago Naples New York Philadelphia Portland
London Madrid Mexico City Singapore Sydney Tokyo Toronto Wiesbaden

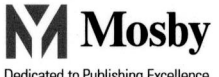

Mosby

Dedicated to Publishing Excellence

Publisher: Nancy Coon
Senior Editor: Sally Schrefer
Developmental Editor: Gail Brower
Project Manager: Dana Peick
Senior Production Editor: Catherine Albright
Manufacturing Supervisor: Karen Lewis
Designer: Jeanne Wolfgeher
Cover Designer: Amy Buxton

Printing/Binding by Western Publishing

Printed in the United States of America

Mosby-Year Book, Inc.
11830 Westline Industrial Drive
St. Louis, Missouri 63146

ISBN 0-8151-8024-1
27056

95 96 97 98 99   /   9 8 7 6 5 4 3 2 1

■ ACKNOWLEDGMENTS

I wish to express my appreciation to the physicians, nurse reviewers, and consultants who gave their time and expertise in their areas of specialty:

William Honigman, MD
Diplomate, American Board of Emergency Medicine
Emergency Department Kaiser Permanente,
Anaheim, California

Stephen J. Munz, MD
Diplomate, American Board of Ophthalmology
Eye Physician and Surgeon
Kaiser Permanente, Anaheim, California

Nancy Perkins, MSN, RN, CS Clinical Nurse Specialist
Department of Psychiatry
Kaiser Permanente, Anaheim, California

Mary Jo Shaffer, MD
Obstetrics & Gynecology
Kaiser Permanente, La Palma, California

Minoru Yoshida, MD, FAAP
Infants, Children, and Adolescents
Kaiser Permanente, Anaheim, California

I also wish to thank Phyllis Gallagher, JD, RN, for her guidance and insight into the potential legal issues related to telephone triage.

Thank you to the wonderful telephone triage nurses at Kaiser Permanente whom I have had the opportunity to work with. Thanks to all who have participated in my research projects and have offered helpful suggestions, expert advice, and mental and emotional support through trying times!

■ DEDICATION

This book is dedicated to those who listen, guide, and compassionately care for the patients and parents who call them for help and advice.

CONTENTS

■ INTRODUCTION

When a patient calls with a health problem, do you always know the appropriate questions to ask? Do you ask direct questions that will first rule out a serious condition (primary assessment)? Do you then continue with questions in a simple and systematic but comprehensive fashion (secondary assessment)? Telephone triage is not new; yet, there are few resources that provide the guidance and tools needed to perform an appropriate and comprehensive telephone assessment.

Telephone Health Assessment: Guidelines for Practice contains guidelines for interviewing and triaging the patient with an acute health care problem or concern. It contains "fingertip" information in a user-friendly format. Guidelines for telephone health assessment are based on the caller's identified problem and on the body system or area of the body the caller is concerned with. At times, the caller may not "fit" into any one assessment guideline, or the health complaint may be vague, varied, and multiple. It may not be possible to use a single assessment. The utmost caution and care should be given to these patients. These guidelines are not intended for use with the individual with chronic or multiple health problems, nor is this book intended to be a "cookbook" for health screening or medical advice.

Telephone triage has been defined as the process of collecting information over the telephone to determine the urgency of a health problem and to determine whether medical intervention is needed and how soon treatment should begin. The level of urgency is categorized according to the individual's need for intervention. The American Hospital Association classifies a medical problem in one of the following categories:*

Emergent:	• Condition requires immediate medical attention.
	• Delay is harmful to the individual.
	• Disorder is acute and is potentially a threat to life or function.
Urgent:	• Condition requires medical attention within a few hours.
	• Patient is in danger if not attended.
	• Disorder is acute but not severe.
Nonurgent:	• Condition does not require emergency service.
	• Disorder is minor or nonacute.

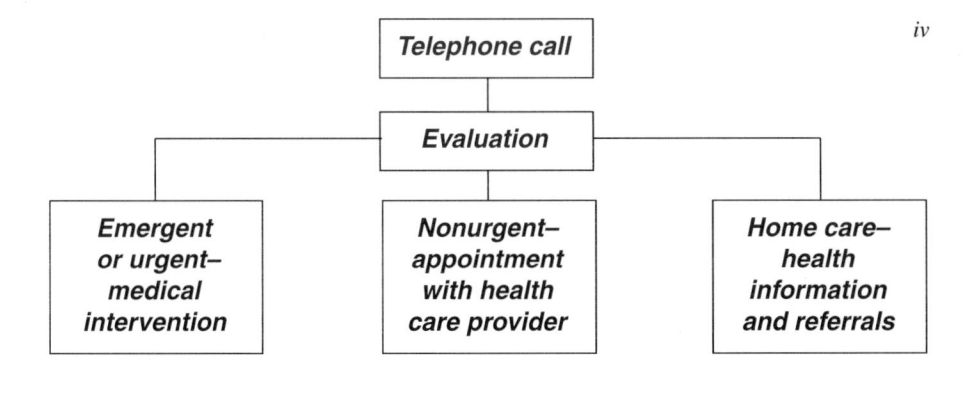

These guidelines are written for nurses who have an extensive medical-surgical background and experience in obstetrics, gynecology, pediatrics, and in the emergency room or intensive care unit. Such individuals have an understanding of the significance of the recommended questioning and the consequences of the caller's response to the questioning. The specific assessment and triage guidelines are intended to provide those receiving these calls with appropriate comprehensive questioning; yet, these questions encourage the use of professional experience and good judgment when recommending specific interventions. Usually the user will not need to complete all the questions during the interview before recommending interventions. In fact, emergency interventions need to be made as soon as possible after it is determined that an emergency situation exists. If an appointment is appropriate, the user should determine how soon the patient should be seen, in what type of setting the patient should be seen, and, in some cases, what type of health care provider is most appropriate. Some home care instructions for common health problems are also included.

The user accepts full responsibility for emergency and other interventions, as well as when, and if, during the telephone interview, they are appropriate.

The medical problems listed are intended to assist the telephone interviewer and, perhaps, trigger more specific questioning. It is not the intention of this text to suggest that the person using these guidelines make a medical diagnosis; rather, this book is written to help the user understand the potential gravity of each patient's situation.

*Mancini M, Gale AT: *Emergency care and the law*, Rockville, Aspen System, 1981, per McGear R, Simms J, 1988.

TELEPHONE CONSULTATION FORM

ⅣⅣ Mosby

Name _John Doe_   Birth Date _2-16-35_   Date _7-1-95_

Phone _222-333-4444_   Call Received _10³⁰_ (AM) _____ PM

Health Care Provider _Dr. Scott_

1. CHIEF COMPLAINT or CONCERN _" Chest tightness "_

Onset _X 3 hours_

2. NURSING ASSESSMENT _Constant, mild substernal - scale 1-3_
" I don't think it's anything." " She made me call."
Wife present. Mild "tingling" of ℝ arm X 10 min.

☐ Temperature _N/A_	☐ Sore Throat _____
☐ Rash	☐ Swollen Glands _____
☐ Cough _none_	☐ Ear Ache _____
☐ Congestion _none_	☐ Body Aches _____
☐ Chest Pain _denies_	☐ Abdominal Pain _N/A_
☑ Short of Breath _slight_	☐ Nausea _____ ☐ Vomiting _____
☑ Sweating _mild_	☐ Diet _____
☑ Dizziness _slight on + off_	☐ Appetite: Poor / Good _____
☑ Indigestion _p̄ breakfast @ 7 AM_	☐ Diarrhea _____
☑ Weakness _mild_	☐ Constipation _____
☐ Left Arm or Other Pain _denies_	☐ Urination: Painful / Frequent / Urgent _____

Health History _Hypertension_

Medications _Zestril_

Allergies _N/A_

L.M.P. _N/A_   Birth Control Method _N/A_

Immunizations / Last Tetanus _N/A_

3. NURSING INTERVENTIONS / ADVICE _911_

10⁴⁵/AM Call back by nurse.
Wife states paramedics just arrived

DISPOSITIONS: ☑ 911   ☐ Appointment _____
        ☐ Advice   ☐ ER _____
        ☐ Referral(s) _____

Instructions Accepted   Yes ☑   No ☐
Noncompliance Warning   Yes ☑ _Strong cardiac_
If S/S Increase (or No Improvement) Call Back for: _N/A_

Nurse's Signature _Sandra Simonsen R.N., M.S.N._

■ **DOCUMENTING TELEPHONE ASSESSMENT**

Documentation provides a complete patient record, promotes communication between all members of the health care team, validates nursing practice, and provides legal protection for the patient, nurse, and health care facility. Using appropriate forms and guidelines provides structure for comprehensive documentation of the telephone consultation. This sample form documents the patient-nurse telephone consultation.

CARDIAC ASSESSMENT

WHAT IS THE MAIN PROBLEM OR CONCERN?

How severe is it (on a scale from 0 to 5)?   When did it begin?   How is the patient responding?   Is the patient alone?

■ PAIN

Describe the pain or discomfort. Is there a feeling of heaviness, pressure, or tightness in the chest? Is the pain sharp? Can the pain be described as crushing or vicelike?

What is the exact location of the pain (midsternal)?

Does the pain or discomfort radiate to the jaw, shoulder, arm, or back?

Is there a tingling or numbness in the jaw, arm, back, or shoulder?

Does it hurt to press the area(s) of pain?

Is the pain worse on inspiration or expiration?

■ ACCOMPANYING SIGNS AND SYMPTOMS

Is there shortness of breath?

Is there a blue or gray discoloration in the fingernail beds, lips, or earlobes?

Is the patient sweating?

Is there a feeling of weakness, dizziness, or faintness?

Is there indigestion, heartburn, or nausea?

Is there cough or congestion?

Is there leg pain, edema, or redness?

Are the ankles swollen?

Are there any factors that aggravate or relieve the symptoms?

■ HISTORY

Is there a history of angina, congestive heart failure, heart attack, or problem with an irregular heart beat?

Is there a history of blood clotting problems?

Does the patient smoke?

What medications, prescribed and over-the-counter, is the patient taking?

POSSIBLE MEDICAL PROBLEMS

Angina–stable	Atelectasis	Gallbladder colic	Mitral valve prolapse	Pulmonary edema or embolism
Angina–unstable	Congenital heart disease	Gastroesophageal reflux or spasm	Myocardial infarction	Rhythmic disorders
Anxiety	Costochrondritis	Hiatal hernia	Pericarditis	Ruptured aortic aneurysm
Aortic aneurysm	Endocarditis	Lung abscess	Pneumothorax	Upper respiratory infection or bronchitis

TRIAGE GUIDELINES

▶ Call 911, Paramedics, or ER if:	▶ Make same-day appointment if:	▶ Call back for appointment if:
• Chest pain, tightness, or pressure develops, especially if accompanied by shortness of breath, sweating, dizziness, or indigestion	• Chest pain persists without other significant signs and symptoms occurring over a more extended period of time • Chest pain is not present at the time of the telephone call	• Chest pain reoccurs • Significant signs or symptoms reoccur (shortness of breath, dizziness, sweating, nausea or indigestion, significant weakness, or pain in the left arm, shoulder, upper abdomen, neck, or jaw)

⬣ PRECAUTIONS

- Be aware of the possible "denial of heart attack" phenomenon.
- Assume that the chest pain is cardiac related until proven otherwise.
- Be aware that cardiac pain may or may not radiate to the shoulder, jaw, or teeth, and may not travel down the left or right arm, back, or upper abdomen. Chest pain may be totally absent with the individual reporting vague indigestion, weakness, or other symptoms.
- Send paramedics if you think the situation may be life threatening.
- Always choose the cautious alternative.
- Specifically caution the patient against driving or being driven by another to a medical facility. Strong cardiac noncompliant warnings are indicated. For example, "If you are having a heart attack, it is dangerous to drive to the hospital; you could faint or die in route."
- According to the American Heart Association, more than one half of all heart attack patients die outside the hospital, most within 2 hours of the initial symptoms.

🏠 HOME CARE INSTRUCTIONS

There are no Home Care Instructions for chest pain.

RESPIRATORY ASSESSMENT

WHAT IS THE MAIN PROBLEM OR CONCERN?

How severe is it (on a scale from 0 to 5)?   When did it begin?   How is the patient responding?   Is the patient alone?

■ RESPIRATORY CHARACTERISTICS

Is the patient able to speak?
Is there nasal flaring, or are the neck muscles used to breathe?
Is the patient unable to breathe when lying down?
Is there a blue or gray discoloration in the fingernail beds, lips, or earlobes?
Is the patient sweating? Is the skin hot or cold?
Is there cough or congestion?
What color is the sputum? Is blood present?
What is the respiratory rate?
Are there any factors that aggravate or relieve the symptoms?

Pediatric considerations:

Is there a possibility or history of swallowed objects?
Does the chest "suck in" when the child inhales?
Is respiration noisy? Is the rate rapid?
Is excess drooling evident? Is the child able to swallow?
Is the child eating or drinking? Is vomiting or diarrhea present?
Is there a "barky" cough? Is there a history of croup or asthma?

■ CHEST PAIN OR DISCOMFORT

Describe the pain or discomfort. Is there a feeling of heaviness, pressure, or tightness in the chest? Is the pain sharp?
How severe is the pain (on a scale from 0 to 5)?
What is the exact location of the pain?

Is the pain worse on inspiration or expiration?
Does it hurt to press the areas of pain?
Does the pain or discomfort radiate to the jaw, shoulder, arms, or back?
Is there indigestion, heartburn, or nausea?

■ ACCOMPANYING SIGNS AND SYMPTOMS

Is there a feeling of weakness, dizziness, or faintness?
Is there nasal congestion? If so, what is the color of the nasal discharge?
Is there pain, swelling, or redness in the legs?
Is there fever?
Is there throat, ear, or facial pain?
Is there headache or body ache?
Has there been previous stress or anxiety?

■ HISTORY

Has there been recent trauma, surgery, diagnostic procedure, or hospitalization? What medications does the individual take?
Are there chronic health conditions?
Is there a history of breathing problems–asthma, emphysema, pneumonia, or tuberculosis?
Is there a history of positive HIV status or congestive heart failure?
Has there been a recent exposure to environmental irritants?
Does the individual smoke?
Are there any known allergies?

POSSIBLE MEDICAL PROBLEMS

Anaphylaxis	Botulism	Diabetic ketoacidosis	Pneumothorax	*Pediatric:* Asthma
Aspiration or choking	Bronchitis	Influenza syndrome	Pulmonary embolism	Broncholitis
Asthma	Chronic obstructive pulmonary disease	Pleurisy	Respiratory arrest	Epiglottiditis
Atelectasis	Congestive heart failure	Pneumonia		Gastroenteritis with dehydration

TRIAGE GUIDELINES

▶ Call 911, Paramedics, or ER if:

- Breathing has ceased
- Severe respiratory distress exists
- Foreign body inhibits breathing
- Noisy, difficult breathing develops
- Blue or gray discoloration of finger nail beds, lips, or earlobes exists
- Skin is cool and moist to the touch
- Chest pain or discomfort develops

Pediatric considerations:

- Excessive irritability or lethargy, inability to eat or drink (swallow), fever, rapid noisy breathing, retraction, wheezing, or blue or gray discoloration of skin, lips, or earlobes persists

▶ Make same-day appointment if:

- Onset of mild or moderate shortness of breath gradually persists
- Noisy breathing or severe cough develops without significant difficulty in breathing, without chest pain or dizziness, and without blue or gray discoloration of fingernail beds, lips, or earlobes

▶ Call back for appointment if:

- Respiratory signs or symptoms increase or do not improve with home care instructions
- Chest, shoulder, neck, or upper abdominal pain develops; dizziness, weakness, nausea, sweating, or significant weakness persists
- Severe nasal or head congestion is not relieved with over-the-counter medications
- Earache or facial pain develops
- Severe nasal or head congestion persists
- Fever of 102° or above develops over 48 hr
- Severe cough persists
- Yellow, green, or brown nasal discharge persists for several days
- Green, brown, or blood-tinged sputum appears
- Sore throat does not improve with home care
- Exposed to Strep throat
- Individual appears or acts extremely ill

⬤ PRECAUTIONS

- Always send paramedics if you think the situation may be life threatening.
- Specifically caution the patient against driving or being driven by another to a medical facility. The patient may die in route.
- Always be cautious, and recommend the safer alternative.
- When sending the patient for medical assessment, consider whether the facility has the ability to assess arterial blood gases or provide mechanical ventilation.

Pre-ER Instructions:

- ➤ Instruct patient to sit to decrease energy expenditure and to assist breathing.
- ➤ Calm and reassure the caller.
- ➤ Prepare to give emergency instructions on respiratory or cardiopulmonary assessment and, if necessary, CPR instructions or the Heimlich maneuver to a family member.

🏠 HOME CARE INSTRUCTIONS *(for uncomplicated cough or nasal congestion of recent onset)*

Advise the patient that viruses may last 7 to 10 days, that antibiotics do not cure colds or influenza, and that over-the-counter medications are available for relief of symptoms and fever. (Check with health care provider.)

1. Rest at home.
2. If not restricted, drink plenty of fluids, preferably warm or hot, not iced.
3. Use vaporizer to thin secretions and soothe nasal and respiratory passageways.
4. Keep room temperature at 65° or lower. A hot, dry environment will increase the congestion of the nose and head.
5. Avoid exposure to smoke, wind, dust, and smog.
6. If additional signs or symptoms develop, or if the patient does not improve daily, instruct the patient to call back for further assessment.

GASTROINTESTINAL ASSESSMENT

WHAT IS THE MAIN PROBLEM OR CONCERN?

How severe is it (on a scale from 0 to 5)?   When did it begin?   How is the patient responding?

■ GASTROINTESTINAL CHARACTERISTICS

Describe the pain or discomfort. Is the pain sharp, dull, or throbbing?
What is the exact location of the pain?
Is the area tender to pressure or to the touch?
How severe is the pain (on a scale from 0 to 5)?
Is it constant or intermittent?
Does it radiate to other areas?
Is there distention or flatus?
Are there any factors that aggravate or relieve the symptoms?

Pediatric considerations:

Is the child drawing up his or her legs and crying?
Can the child be calmed?
Describe the eating and sleeping patterns.
Is there vomiting, diarrhea, or constipation?
Is there blood in the stool?

■ ACCOMPANYING SIGNS AND SYMPTOMS

Is there vomiting? If so, what is the frequency and characteristics (fecal odor, bloody, or coffee ground)?
Is there constipation or diarrhea? If so, what is the frequency and characteristics (light in color or tarry; presence of blood or mucus)?
Is there indigestion or heartburn?

Is there urine output? If so, is the frequency at least once every 8 hours?
Are there signs or symptoms of dehydration (dry mucous membranes, decreased urine output and dark color, sunken eyes, weakness, and lethargy)?

Pediatric considerations:

Are there tears when the child or infant cries?
If the patient is an infant, is the fontanelle sunken?
Is there fever? Is there jaundice?

■ HISTORY

What has been the recent intake of food, fluids, or alcohol?
Has there been recent trauma or major stress? Has there been recent abdominal or other surgery, diagnostic procedure, or hospitalization?
Are there any chronic health conditions or a history of gastrointestinal bleeding?
If the patient is a woman, when was the last menstrual period? What method of birth control is the patient using?
If the patient is a child, is there a possibility or history of swallowing objects?
Has there been recent travel out of the country? Have there been recent camping trips?
Has there been use of antibiotics in the past 6 weeks?
What medications, prescribed and over-the-counter, is the patient taking?

POSSIBLE MEDICAL PROBLEMS

Aneurysm	Dysmenorrhea	Hepatitis	Pelvic inflammatory disease	Congenital intestinal atresia or
Appendicitis	Ectopic pregnancy	Hiatal hernia	Peptic ulcer	stenosis
Cholecystitis	Flatulence	Indigestion	Renal calculi	Incarcerated hernia
Constipation or dehydration	Food poisoning, Salmonella, *Shigella*	Intestinal obstruction	Urinary tract infection	Intussusception
Diabetic ketoacidosis	Gastroenteritis, gastritis, and colitis	Irritable bowel syndrome	*Pediatric:*	Necrotizing enterocolitis
Diverticular disease	Gastroesophageal reflux	Pancreatitis	Colic	Pyloric stenosis

TRIAGE GUIDELINES

▶ Call 911, Paramedics, or ER if:

- Severe weakness, lethargy, or faintness occurs because of fluid loss from vomiting or diarrhea
- Stool is grossly bloody
- Severe abdominal pain persists

Pediatric considerations:
- Child or infant refuses fluids and is showing obvious signs of dehydration (moderate to severe lethargy, leathery skin, no tears when crying, dry mucous membranes, sunken eyes, and urine output <q8hr)
- A history of recent head injury exists
- Parent is unable to calm uncontrolled crying
- Patient has a stiff neck with fever
- Rapid breathing develops

▶ Make same-day appointment if:

- Vomiting and diarrhea is uncontrolled without a response to home care instructions
- Abdominal pain persists
- Blood in stool appears

Pediatric considerations:
- Child or infant refuses fluids and is showing mild to moderate signs of dehydration

▶ Call back for appointment if:

- Vomiting continues >2hr
- Signs and symptoms of dehydration increase (dry mucous membranes [mouth], dizziness, significant weakness, urine output is <q8hr, or sunken eyes)
- Severe diarrhea persists without improvement >4hr
- Mucus or blood in the stool exists
- Abdominal pain, high fever, or lethargy develops
- Patient acts and looks extremely ill

CAUTION: THE YOUNGER THE CHILD–THE FASTER DEHYDRATION MAY OCCUR

⬡ PRECAUTIONS

- If the individual is a diabetic patient, consider that a hypoglycemic reaction is possible. Diabetic acidosis may be life threatening.
- Tarry-black stools or coffee ground emesis may indicate internal bleeding. Pepto Bismol or iron supplements may also cause tarry-black stools.
- When sending the patient for medical assessment, consider whether the facility can provide intravenous fluid replacement and has a laboratory equipped to provide immediate electrolyte evaluation.

🏠 HOME CARE INSTRUCTIONS *(for adults: vomiting and diarrhea)*

1. Consume nothing by mouth 60 minutes after the last episode of vomiting.
2. Begin with sips of warm, clear liquids (clear broth, Jello, Kool Aid, water, and weak tea) and electrolyte-replacement drinks (Gatorade) in the first 12 hours. Increase fluids to tolerance. For the next 12 hours, add small amounts of white rice, apple sauce, banana, toast, pretzels, soda crackers, or baked potato (no milk or butter).
3. If there are no signs of improvement within 2 to 4 hours or if signs or symptoms increase, call back for further assessment and instructions.

4. If the individual is not voiding at least once in 8 hours, make an appointment for evaluation.
5. Gradually introduce additional bland foods during the next 1 to 2 days. Do not return to a normal diet for 4 to 5 days.
6. If high fever or abdominal pain develops, call for an appointment.

Pediatric home care instructions *(for vomiting and diarrhea)*

- Nothing by mouth for 30 minutes after the last episode of vomiting.
- For infants: begin introducing Pedialyte, Ricelyte, or Lytrin (1 tbsp every 10 to 15 minutes). Increase fluids to tolerance.
- For older infants (who normally have juices) and children: introduce Gatorade or other electrolyte-replacement fluids (1 tbsp every 10 to 15 minutes), then other clear fluids as tolerated for age, such as water, broth, Kool Aid, Jello, and Popsicles. Increase fluids to tolerance.
- Breast-feeding infants may resume after 4 to 6 hours; formula-fed infants may resume with half water–half formula after 4 to 6 hours; milk-fed children may return to full strength after 12 to 24 hours.
- Keep on bland diet for 2 to 3 days; return to normal diet as child allows.

ABDOMINAL PAIN ASSESSMENT

WHAT IS THE MAIN PROBLEM OR CONCERN?

How severe is it (on a scale from 0 to 5)?   What is the location of the pain?   Is the patient alone?

■ ABDOMINAL CHARACTERISTICS

Is the individual doubled over or drawing up his or her legs?
Describe the characteristics of the pain (sharp, dull, or throbbing).
When did the pain begin?
Describe the activity when the pain was first noted.
Does the pain radiate to the back, pelvis, or chest?
Is the pain constant or intermittent?
Are there areas that are tender to the touch?
Is there a bulge or lump in the abdomen or groin?

Pediatric considerations:

Is the infant drawing up his or her legs and crying?
Can the child be calmed?
Is there a history of colic? Are there "fussy" times in the afternoon or evening?
Is there fever, vomiting, diarrhea, or constipation?
What is the activity pattern of the child?
Is the child eating and drinking?
Does the child appear and act sick?
Does the pain appear to be mild or severe (on a scale from 0 to 5)?
Is there a history of swallowed objects?
Has there been a change in the child's breathing pattern?
Does the child urinate frequently? Does it appear to be painful?

■ ACCOMPANYING SIGNS AND SYMPTOMS

Is distention of the abdomen or flatus present?
Is there indigestion or heartburn?
Is there vomiting? If so, what is the frequency and characteristics (fecal odor, bloody, or vomitus coffee ground)?
Is there constipation or diarrhea? If so, what is the frequency and characteristics? (Is the stool light in color? Is blood or mucus present?)
Is there dysuria or a frequency of urination? Is the urine dark?
Is there urine output? If so, is the frequency at least once every 8 hours?
Is there fever?
Is jaundice present?

■ HISTORY

What has been the recent intake of food, fluids, and alcohol?
Has there been recent trauma or major stress? Has there been recent abdominal or other surgery, diagnostic procedure, or hospitalization?
If the patient is a woman, when was the last menstrual period? What method of birth control is the patient using?
Has there been recent travel out of the country or camping trips?
Are there any chronic conditions, especially of the gastrointestinal system?
Is there a history of abdominal pain?
What medications, prescribed and over-the-counter, is the patient taking?

POSSIBLE MEDICAL PROBLEMS

Aneurysm	Diabetic ketoacidosis	Gastroenteritis	Intestinal obstruction	*Salmonella*	*Pediatric:*
Appendicitis	Diverticular disease	Gastroesophageal reflux	Irritable bowel syndrome	Trauma–hematoma	Colic
Cholecystitis	Dysmenorrhea	Gastritis	Lactose intolerance	Tumor–mass	Congenital intestinal atresia or stenosis
Colitis	Ectopic pregnancy	Hepatitis	Peptic ulcer	Urinary tract infec-	Incarcerated hernia
Constipation	Flatulence	Hiatal hernia	Renal calculi	tion	Intussusception
Dehydration	Food poisoning	Indigestion	Pelvic inflammatory disease		Necrotizing enterocolitis

TRIAGE GUIDELINES

▶ Call 911, Paramedics, or ER if:	▶ Make same-day appointment if:	▶ Call back for appointment if:
• Severe abdominal pain persists, especially if the patient has other significant signs and symptoms that include high fever, persistent vomiting, severe diarrhea, weakness, dizziness, fainting, prefainting sensation, or severe lethargy • History of recent head injury exists	• Moderate abdominal pain develops • Mild abdominal pain persists	• Pain increases or if there is no improvement with home care instructions • Other significant signs and symptoms develop

⬤ PRECAUTIONS

- If the patient is a woman of childbearing age, consider ectopic pregnancy, a life-threatening condition.
- For the pregnant woman with abdominal pain, refer the patient to an obstetrics professional.
- If pain is severe, consume nothing by mouth before medical assessment.
- If the individual is in severe pain, recommend that a family member or friend drive the patient to a medical facility.
- When sending the patient for medical assessment for abdominal pain, consider whether the facility has the ability to provide immediate testing for pregnancy; complete blood count with sedimentation rate, blood urea nitrogen, urine and serum amylase, blood sugar; and urine analysis with culture and sensitivity.
- If the patient has a chronic illness with frequent episodes of abdominal pain and if the signs and symptoms are worse than usual, recommend that the patient contact the health care provider who has previously treated the condition.

Pediatric considerations:

- If the child has suffered a recent injury or could have swallowed an object, recommend that the patient be seen by a health care provider.
- If child is looking or acting ill or is complaining of persistent abdominal pain, he or she should be seen by a health care provider.

🏠 HOME CARE INSTRUCTIONS

For adult with mild abdominal pain:

1. A warm bath or a heating pad on low heat placed on the abdominal area for 20 to 30 minutes may provide relief. Call for an appointment if there is no relief or if the pain or discomfort increases.
2. Consume clear liquids, and maintain a bland diet until symptoms resolve.
3. If constipated, caution the patient against taking laxatives.

For child with colic:

1. Colic is not serious; however, it is frustrating for a parent. An infant with colic is under 3 months of age. Instruct parent to take child's temperature. If any fever is present, child should be seen immediately by a health care provider.
2. Suggestions for calming child:
   - ➤ Take child for a ride in the car.
   - ➤ Have child listen to constant noises (refrigerator humming, fish tank motor).
   - ➤ Have child feel gentle vibrations. (Put baby in infant seat on top of running clothes dryer.)

9

MUSCULOSKELETAL ASSESSMENT

WHAT IS THE MAIN PROBLEM OR CONCERN?

How severe is the pain (on a scale from 0 to 5)?   If there is an injury, is a bone protruding, or is there an obvious deformity (out of alignment)?
When did the problem begin?   How is the patient responding?

■ PAIN

Describe the activity when the pain was first noted.
What is the exact location of the pain?
Does the pain or discomfort radiate to other areas?
Are there activities or positions that aggravate or relieve the symptoms?
Is there motor impairment, numbness, tingling, or paralysis?
Are there changes in skin color? If so, describe color.
If the area of pain or injury is a limb, is there a pulse distal to the affected area?

■ LEG PAIN

What is the exact location of the pain?
Describe the size of the affected area.
Is there swelling?
Is there redness?
Is it tender to touch the area?

■ HISTORY

Has there been a recent injury?
Is there a history of gout?
Is there a history of arthritis?
Is there a history of neuromuscular disease?
Is there a history of hypokalemia? Is the patient taking diuretics?
Is there a history of thrombophlebitis or pulmonary embolism?
Is there a history of cardiovascular disease or other chronic condition?
Has there been recent prolonged inactivity?
Is the patient using medication for any condition?

POSSIBLE MEDICAL PROBLEMS		
Arthritis	Dislocation or subluxation	Osteomyelitis
Bone fracture	Gout	Thrombophlebitis
Bursitis	Guillain-Barré syndrome	Torn tendon
Claudication	Muscle spasm, strain, or sprain	

TRIAGE GUIDELINES

▶ Call 911, Paramedics, or ER if:	▶ Make same-day appointment if:	▶ Call back for appointment if:
• Severe injury or severe pain exists • Limb, finger, or toe develops a pale or blue color when compared with other skin tones • Absence of a distal pulse in the injured or painful limb exists	• Patient is unable to function normally with muscular or skeletal signs or symptoms • Leg pain persists with redness or edema	• Muscular or skeletal signs or symptoms do not improve with home care instructions • Other significant signs or symptoms develop

⬤ PRECAUTIONS *(for severe injuries)*

- Patient should not be moved.
- Immobilize affected area, if possible. Movement may cause damage to the spinal cord or major arteries and nerves. The elderly patient may have a hip fracture. Caution should be taken if the patient has fallen and is experiencing hip, leg, or lower back pain.
- Severe neck or back injury may be a threat to life and future functioning.
- Consider shock in all cases of trauma.
- Rib fractures may cause lung or kidney injuries.
- A fracture of the pelvis may lead to bruising or rupturing of the bladder.
- If thrombophlebitis (red, warm, and tender area of leg) is suspected, avoid rubbing or applying pressure to the affected area. Make appointment as soon as possible, or come to the emergency room.

Precautions for limb trauma:

- Any injury without a pulse in the distal area, any malalignment of an extremity, or any pale or blue discoloration of the skin distal to the injury should be seen immediately by a health care provider. Immediate medical attention may be necessary to save the patient's life or limb.

Pre-ER Instructions (for severed part)

- ➤ Wrap severed part in a wet gauze or towel.
- ➤ Place part in a sealed plastic bag and place bag inside a second plastic bag. Fill the outer bag with crushed ice.

🏠 HOME CARE INSTRUCTIONS *(for minor injury)*

1. Immobilize and elevate area of injury. Do not walk on sprained ankle.
2. Apply cool, moist compress to the injured area for the first 24 hours.
3. Apply support (Ace bandage) if there is an injured joint.
4. Over-the-counter medication should be taken for mild pain. (Check with a health care provider.)
5. Apply a warm moist compress after 24 hours.
6. If there is no improvement in 24 to 48 hours or if other signs or symptoms develop, call for an appointment with a health care provider.

HEAD INJURY ASSESSMENT

WHAT IS THE MAIN PROBLEM OR CONCERN?

If there is an open injury, is bleeding under control?   What is the current level of consciousness?   When did the injury occur?   Is the patient alone?

■ TRAUMA

What was the severity of the impact?
What is the size and location of the affected area?
Has the patient experienced loss of consciousness? If so, for how long?
Does the patient have normal orientation to time and place?
Does the patient exhibit unusual behavior? Is there confusion or lethargy?
Is the patient able to move arms or legs normally?
Are pupils equal and reactive to light?
Are there visual changes?
Is there vomiting?
Is there drainage from the ears or nose?
Is there fever?

■ HISTORY

What is the nature of the trauma (abuse or assault)?
Have there been other recent illnesses?
Is there drug or alcohol use?
Is the patient using medications for any condition?
If it is an open injury, when was the last tetanus booster?

POSSIBLE MEDICAL PROBLEMS

Concussion	Skull fracture
Contusion	(depressed)
Intracranial bleeding	Subdural hematoma

TRIAGE GUIDELINES

▶ Call 911, Paramedics, or ER if:	▶ Make same-day appointment if:	▶ Call back for appointment if:
• Massive or severe head injury or head injury with a loss of consciousness has occurred • Blood or fluid drains from the ears or nose • Repeated vomiting, severe lethargy, or a weakness of extremities develop • Pupils are unequal or visual changes occur • Unusual behavior (agitation or confusion) develops • Abnormal breathing pattern exists	• Minor to moderate head injury requires sutures without significant other signs or symptoms • Patient needs tetanus booster	• Health status changes (see note under Precautions)

⬢ PRECAUTIONS

- To stop bleeding, hold a cool wet cloth directly to area with firm pressure for 10 to 15 minutes.
- If there is a loss of consciousness, the patient should seek medical assessment; consider whether the recommended facility has the ability to perform a CAT scan, if necessary.
- Instruct the patient to go to the emergency room if any of the following signs or symptoms develop:
  - ➤ Unusual behavior such as agitation or disorientation
  - ➤ Drainage of fluid or blood from the ears or nose
  - ➤ Unequal pupils or difficulty seeing
  - ➤ Repeated vomiting
  - ➤ Change in respiratory rate (labored or sporadic)
- Always recommend a driver to the emergency room.

🏠 HOME CARE INSTRUCTIONS *(for mild head injury)*

1. Apply cool compresses to the area of injury for 2 hours.
2. Arouse the patient every 2 hours to check alertness and orientation; monitor for the next 24 hours.
3. Maintain a light diet.
4. Activities should remain quiet.

HEADACHE ASSESSMENT

WHAT IS THE MAIN PROBLEM OR CONCERN?

What is the severity of the pain (on a scale from 0 to 5)? When did it begin? How is the patient responding? Is the patient alone?

■ PAIN

What is the exact location of the pain?
Has there been a change in the level of consciousness, orientation, or behavior?
Are there visual changes?
Is there nausea or vomiting?
Is there fever? If so, how high?
Is there stiffness in the neck?
Is there an inability to move the head freely or to touch the chin to the chest?
What, if anything, has already been done to try to relieve the pain?

■ HISTORY

Is there a history of headaches (migraine, cluster, stress related)?
Is there sinus congestion?
Is there a toothache or other dental problem?
Has there been a recent injury?
Is there a major life change or stress?
Is the patient taking any medications?
Are there any chronic health conditions?

POSSIBLE MEDICAL PROBLEMS

Cluster headache	Migraine headache
Dental abscess	Sinusitis
Dental infection	Stress-related headache
Encephalitis	Subarachnoid hemorrhage

TRIAGE GUIDELINES

▶ Call 911, Paramedics, or ER if:	▶ Make same-day appointment if:	▶ Call back for appointment if:
• Severe headache ("Worst I've ever had.") persists with or without neck stiffness, fever, and nausea and vomiting • Disorientation, agitation, or lethargy develops	• Moderate to severe headache exists without other significant signs or symptoms • Patient has a history of migraine headaches	• Headache pain continues without improvement with home care instructions • Other significant signs or symptoms develop

⬣ PRECAUTIONS

- If patient describes headache as "the worst in my life," consider subarachnoid hemorrhage. This condition is life threatening.

🏠 HOME CARE INSTRUCTIONS *(for headache without other significant signs and symptoms)*

1. Apply a cool compress to the head.
2. Rest in dark, quiet room.
3. Take an over-the-counter analgesic after checking with a health care provider.
4. If headache does not improve in 1 to 2 hours, recommend that the patient call back for an appointment with a health care provider.

15

NEUROLOGIC ASSESSMENT

WHAT IS THE MAIN PROBLEM OR CONCERN?

How severe is it (on a scale from 0 to 5)?   When did it begin?   How is the patient responding?   Is the patient alone?

■ NEUROLOGIC CHARACTERISTICS

Did the problem begin suddenly or gradually?

Is the condition getting better or worse, or is it the same since its onset?

What is the current level of orientation?

Has there been a recent trauma?

Has there been a loss of consciousness? If so, for how long?

Have there been changes in the speech pattern?

Is there a facial droop or drooling?

Is there weakness of the extremities?

Is there numbness or tingling?

Has there been a loss of bowel or bladder control?

Are there visual changes or changes in pupil size?

Is there a change in hearing?

Is there any dizziness or lightheadedness?

Is the patient experiencing tremors, shakiness, or jerky movements?

Is there nausea or vomiting?

■ PAIN

Where is the exact location of the pain?

Describe the severity (on a scale from 0 to 5) and the characteristics of the pain (sharp, dull, or throbbing).

■ HISTORY

Is there a history of seizures?

Is there a history of hypoglycemia, hyperglycemia, or diabetes?

Has there been exposure to chemical agents?

Is there a history of high blood pressure?

What medications, prescribed and over-the-counter, is the patient taking?

Has there been a recent flu immunization?

POSSIBLE MEDICAL PROBLEMS

Cerebral vascular accident   Mononeuritis (Bell's palsy)
Guillain-Barré syndrome   Transient ischemic attack
Meningitis

TRIAGE GUIDELINES

▶ Call 911, Paramedics, or ER if:

- Patient sustains a grand mal seizure (911)
- Patient experiences seizure and is now alert (ER)
- Sudden onset of erratic behavior, dysphasia, or a weakness of limb(s) occurs
- Patient experiences an episode of loss of consciousness
- Pediatric seizure occurs with no fever, or child has a high, uncontrolled fever

▶ Make same-day appointment if:

- There is a gradual onset of mild neurologic signs and symptoms such as tremors, numbness, tingling, forgetfulness, or other behavioral changes
- Face droops without other significant signs and symptoms

Pediatric considerations:

- Patient has experienced a recent seizure with fever; fever is now controlled, and patient is alert

▶ Call back for appointment if:

- Do not advise the patient to call back. Neurologic signs and symptoms should be evaluated by a health care provider.

● **PRECAUTIONS** *(for seizures or convulsions)*

- Protect the patient from injury.
- Roll the individual gently onto his or her left side.
- Check breathing. If the patient is not breathing, refer to CPR guidelines as needed. (Call 911.)
- If the patient has experienced seizure yet has no history of seizure disorder, consider a cardiac event.
- Always recommend a driver if sending the patient to the emergency room.

Pediatric considerations:

- After the seizure, if the child is breathing and is alert and oriented, take his or her temperature rectally or under the arm.
- If temperature is high, lower the fever by Tylenol (after checking with a health care provider). *Do not give a child aspirin.*
- If child is chilled, trembling, or shaking, wrap lower legs and feet in a warm towel or blanket until shaking stops; then give lukewarm bath (trembling and shaking muscles produce more heat). Head and hair should be very wet. Keep the child in bathtub for 30 minutes.
- If the patient does not have a fever, the child should be seen in the emergency room as soon as possible to determine the cause of the seizure.

SKIN ASSESSMENT

WHAT IS THE MAIN PROBLEM OR CONCERN?

How severe is it (on a scale from 0 to 5)?   When did it begin?   How is the patient responding?

■ TRAUMA

What is the extent and type of injury?
Is there bleeding? If so, what is the amount?
Is there impaired range of motion?
If the injury is a laceration, what is the length and depth?
Are sutures required? When was the last tetanus booster?

■ BURNS

Is there redness, blistering, or an involvement of deep tissue?
What is the size of the burn area?

■ PAIN

What is the severity of the pain (on a scale from 0 to 5)?
Are there any factors that aggravate or relieve the pain?

■ RASH

Is the rash flat or elevated?
Are there lesions or blisters?
If there are lesions, how large are they? Do the lesions weep or have
    drainage? Are they all the same size, or do they vary in size?
Is there fever?
Is there vomiting or faintness?
Is itching present? Is there swelling?
Is there numbness or tingling?

■ EXPOSURES

Is there a family member or another with similar signs or symptoms?
Has there been an exposure to poison oak or poison ivy?
Has there been an exposure to a communicable disease?
Has there been an exposure to chemicals?
Has there been an exposure to insect or tick bites?

■ BITES: ANIMAL, HUMAN, AND INSECT

What is the size and location of the area affected?
Is there swelling or redness surrounding the bite? Is there a red streaking?
Is there pain or purulent drainage? Is there fever?
Is a stinger present? If the insect is known, what is its name?
Is there abdominal cramping?
Is there peeling of the skin?

■ HISTORY

Is the patient taking any medications, prescribed or over-the-counter?
Is there a history of allergies?
Has there been recent camping or travel out of the country?
Have there been recent immunizations?
Is there a history of severe allergic reaction to insect stings or bites?
Are there animals in the home?
Does the patient have a sore throat or fever? Is there joint pain?
If the patient is a woman, is menses present? Is there a use of tampons?

POSSIBLE MEDICAL PROBLEMS

Abscess	Cellulitis	Herpes simplex	Infection	Poison oak or ivy	Roseola	Scarlet fever
Allergies	Eczema	Herpes zoster	Lyme disease (if ticks)	Psoriasis	Rubella	Toxic shock syndrome
Anaphylactic reaction	Fifth disease	HIV (if human bite)	Malaria (heat rash)	Rabies (if animal bite)	Rubeola	Varicella
(if insect bite)	Hepatitis (if human bite)	Impetigo	Pediculosis	Ringworm	Scabies	Viral exanthem

TRIAGE GUIDELINES

▶ Call 911, Paramedics, or ER if:

- Patient experiences massive skin injury such as extensive dog bites or burns
- Hives develop with respiratory distress, chest or throat tightness, wheezing or shortness of breath, or difficulty swallowing or speaking
- Hives spread in mouth, tongue, or throat
- Bitten by a black widow or brown recluse spider

▶ Make same-day appointment if:

- Unexplained rash develops
- Unexplained skin lesions develop
- Moderate trauma occurs
- Any trauma occurs if tetanus or booster is due or overdue
- Bitten by a human (HIV and hepatitis B precautions)
- Diabetic with trauma is present
- Hives persists without other significant signs or symptoms

▶ Call back for appointment if:

- Redness, increased pain, swelling, or the presence of pus develops within 24 hours after injury, bite, or burn
- Boil or cyst enlarges or does not open and drain by itself within 24 hours
- Signs or symptoms do not improve with home care instructions

⬤ PRECAUTIONS

- If reaction to insect bites or stings is severe, screen for anaphylaxis and respiratory difficulty (throat or chest tightness, wheezing or shortness of breath, hives, edema, itching).
- With any injury, consider shock.
- For burns, immediately immerse area in cool water for 10 minutes. To cool burn and assist in rehydration of skin tissue, cover with a moist, cool, soft, light dressing.
- If there is a possibility of infectious disease, patient must be isolated in the office or clinic setting.
- If a localized area of redness and pain develops, consider infection, abscess, and cellulitis.
- With any break in skin integrity:
  - ➤ Consider potential for infection.
  - ➤ Use extra caution, if caller is a diabetic patient.
  - ➤ Question the date of the last tetanus booster.
- For insect bites or stings, refer to Home Care Instructions.
- For unidentified rash, refer to "Common Childhood Rashes" on page 46.

🏠 HOME CARE INSTRUCTIONS

For a minor break in skin:

1. Review signs and symptoms of infection with any break in skin integrity.
   - ➤ Redness   ➤ Swelling
   - ➤ Increased pain   ➤ Pus
2. Immediately cleanse area with mild soap and water. Rinse well. If particles are embedded, patient should see a health care provider.
3. Do not apply bandage unless wound is weeping. Bandage or dressing should protect the wound from contamination during the day and should be removed at night to expose the wound to air.
4. Advise the patient on available over-the-counter antibiotic ointments. (Check with health care provider.)

For boils or cysts:

1. Apply warm, moist compresses for 30 minutes, four to five times a day.
2. Caution patient against squeezing or trying to open a boil or cyst.

For insect bites or stings without respiratory distress or rash (if insect is not a black widow or brown recluse spider):

1. Apply paste of $1/_2$ baking soda and $1/_2$ water.
2. Apply a cool, moist compress.
3. Elevate area, if possible.
4. Review signs and symptoms of anaphylaxis and infection listed above. Call back if these develop.

EYE ASSESSMENT

WHAT IS THE MAIN PROBLEM OR CONCERN?

How severe is it (on a scale from 0 to 5)? When did it begin? How is the patient responding? Do the signs and symptoms involve one or both eyes?
What is the location of the signs and symptoms in the eye or visual field?

■ PAIN

Describe the severity (on a scale from 0 to 5) and the characteristics of the pain (sharp, dull, or throbbing).

Are there any factors that aggravate or relieve the pain?

■ ACCOMPANYING SIGNS AND SYMPTOMS

Is there swelling?

Is there tearing?

Is there a discharge or morning crust? If so, what is the color?

Is there redness?

Is there itching or irritation?

Are there visual disturbances (blurring, light flashes, floaters, halos), or is there photosensitivity?

Are the pupils equal in size?

■ HISTORY

Has there been recent trauma? If so, how did it occur?

Have there been any exposures to a foreign body or infection?

Is there a chronic eye condition?

Has there been any previous eye surgery for glaucoma or cataracts?

Does the patient wear glasses or contact lenses?

Is there a history of diabetes?

Is the patient taking any prescribed or over-the-counter medications?

POSSIBLE MEDICAL PROBLEMS

Blepharospasm	Corneal abrasion	Glaucoma–acute	*Newborn:*	Retinal detachment
Cataracts	Corneal laceration	Glaucoma–chronic	Iritis	Retinopathy
Chalazion	Corneal ulcer		Lacrimal obstruction	Stye (external hordeolum)
Conjunctivitis	Foreign body		Nasal obstruction	Vitreal detachment

▶ Call 911, Paramedics, or ER if:	▶ Make same-day appointment if:	▶ Call back for appointment if:
• Perforating or penetrating injury occurs to the eyes • Foreign body or chemical splash enters the eyes (irrigate first) • Pain becomes severe or sudden • Severe loss of visual acuity occurs	• Itching, burning, redness, or colored discharge develops from the eye(s) • Eye pain persists • Loss of visual acuity over a period of time	• Signs and symptoms do not improve with home care instructions • Other significant signs and symptoms develop

⬣ PRECAUTIONS

- If patient reports seeing flashing lights or describes "lightning bolt" visual disturbances, these symptoms may indicate vitreal or retinal detachment. Patient should be seen as soon as possible.
- Visual disturbances may occur as an aura before a headache or may occur in an ocular migraine headache.
- Recommend a driver.

🏠 HOME CARE INSTRUCTIONS

For chemical splash or foreign body in the eye(s):

1. Irrigate eye with lukewarm water for 10 minutes. After irrigation:
   - ➤ Continue to observe, if signs and symptoms or foreign body is gone.
   - ➤ Go to emergency room or call for an appointment if eye pain or irritation persists or particle is not removed by flushing.

For conjunctivitis (pink eye):

1. Use medication as prescribed by a health care provider.
2. Discuss hygiene with the patient to avoid addition of bacteria in eye and to avoid transferring the infection to other individuals.
   - ➤ Wash hands frequently and avoid touching eyes.
   - ➤ Immediately dispose facial tissues after use.
   - ➤ Apply warm moist compresses for comfort, if desired.
   - ➤ Do not allow anyone else to use the same towel or washcloth.

For blood "spot" (subconjunctival hemorrhage) in the sclera of the eye–no pain, injury, or other signs and symptoms:

1. No treatment is needed.
2. Reassure patient that gradual improvement will occur.
3. Notify health care provider if patient is taking Heparin or Coumadin.

For stye (external hordeolum):

1. Apply warm compress to stye for 15 to 20 minutes four to six times per day.
2. If signs or symptoms do not improve in 48 to 72 hours, patient should call back for an appointment with a health care provider.

EAR ASSESSMENT

WHAT IS THE MAIN PROBLEM OR CONCERN?

How severe is it (on a scale from 0 to 5)?   When did it begin?   How is the patient responding?

■ EAR CHARACTERISTICS

What is the location of the pain? External? Internal?
Are there any factors that aggravate or relieve the pain?
Is there swelling or a discharge from the ear?
Is there bleeding?
Is there a hearing loss?
Is there dizziness or ringing in the ears?
Is there redness?

■ ACCOMPANYING SIGNS AND SYMPTOMS

Is there fever?
Is there a sore throat?
Is there nasal congestion?
Is there a headache or facial pain?

■ HISTORY

Is there a history of frequent ear infections?
Is there a history of an ear wax problem?
Is there a history of swimmer's ear?
Has there been trauma (blunt, noise, pressure changes [air travel or mountains])?
Is there a history of using an object (Q-Tip or hair pin) in the ear?
Is the patient taking any prescribed or over-the-counter medications?

POSSIBLE MEDICAL PROBLEMS

Labyrinthitis
Otitis externa
Otitus media
Rupture of eardrum

TRIAGE GUIDELINES

▶ Call 911, Paramedics, or ER if:	▶ Make same-day appointment if:	▶ Call back for appointment if:
• Patient has suffered severe trauma • Foreign body is present (or if there is a history of an object in ear with severe pain)	• Foreign body is present (or if there is a history of object in ear with mild to moderate pain) • Earache persists • Ear discharge develops • There is a history of ear wax problem	Patient with ear signs and symptoms should be evaluated by a health care provider.

⬣ **PRECAUTIONS**

- Hold a cool, moist compress to the ear in cases of severe trauma.
- Any child or adult with a severe earache should be seen by a health care provider as soon as possible. (Eardrum may rupture, which may cause permanent hearing loss as a result of scar tissue.)

- Bloody discharge from the ear may be a result of a rupture of the eardrum.
- If there is a foreign body in the ear, caution against removing it. Make an appointment with a health care professional as soon as possible.

NASAL ASSESSMENT

WHAT IS THE MAIN PROBLEM OR CONCERN?

How severe is it (on a scale from 0 to 5)?   When did it begin?   How is the patient responding?   Is the patient alone?

■ NASAL CHARACTERISTICS

Is there respiratory difficulty?

Can the patient breathe through the mouth without difficulty?

Describe the severity (on a scale from 0 to 5) and the characteristics of the pain (sharp, dull, or throbbing).

Where is the exact location of the pain?

Are there any factors that aggravate or relieve the pain?

Is there bleeding or drainage? If yes, what is the amount?

If there is congestion, what color are the secretions?

Is there swelling?

Is there snoring or difficulty in sleeping?

Is there numbness along the bridge of the nose?

Is there facial pain?

■ ACCOMPANYING SIGNS AND SYMPTOMS

Is there fever?

Is there a sore throat or ear pain?

■ HISTORY

Has there been recent trauma or surgery?

Is a foreign body embedded?

Is there a history of allergies?

Is there nasal drug use?

Is the patient taking prescription or over-the-counter medications?

POSSIBLE MEDICAL PROBLEMS

Allergic rhinitis	Sinusitis
Epistasis	Viral syndrome
Fracture	

TRIAGE GUIDELINES

▶ Call 911, Paramedics, or ER if:	▶ Make same-day appointment if:	▶ Call back for appointment if:
• Patient has suffered a severe trauma • Foreign body is embedded • Nosebleed cannot be controlled by pinching nostrils • Profuse, uncontrolled bleeding develops • Respiratory distress occurs even with mouth breathing	• Green nasal secretions persist • High fever develops • Nosebleed persists (controlled by applied pressure) • Facial pain is present • Earache is present	• Signs and symptoms do not improve with home care instructions • Congestion continues >2 wk

⬢ PRECAUTIONS

- If the patient has suffered a severe trauma, apply cool compress to nose. Breathe through the mouth.
- If foreign body is embedded in the nose, it may fall into respiratory passageways and cause sudden and complete airway obstruction, or it may be aspirated into lungs.

🏠 HOME CARE INSTRUCTIONS

For clear nasal secretions and congestion

1. Adult–Drink 8 to 10 glasses of liquid each day (if not placed on a fluid-restricted diet by a health care provider).
2. Child–Offer fluids frequently, especially clear fluids. Milk should be avoided if it adds to throat congestion.
3. Educate patient about over-the-counter medications for congestion. Check with a health care provider.
4. Infant–Use nasal bulb syringe to gently suction out nose before feeding and before bed.
5. Avoid exposure to smoke and other environmental irritants.
6. A sitting or semi-sitting position provides drainage of nasal and sinus passages.

For nosebleed:

1. Sit up.
2. Pinch soft parts of nose together between thumb and index finger.
3. Breathe through mouth.
4. Hold pinched nose for 10 minutes without letting go.
5. Fill a plastic bag with crushed ice, wrap bag in a towel, and apply to upper nose.
6. Remain sitting in a quiet environment for 30 minutes.
7. Avoid blowing or picking nose (this will remove blood clot, and bleeding will reoccur).
8. Avoid straining or lifting; this may increase pressure, and bleeding will reoccur.
9. Hot, cold, or windy weather may cause drying and crusting of the nasal mucous membranes. Heaters and air conditioners add additional drying to the environment.
10. To prevent nosebleeds:
    - ➤ Use a vaporizer or humidifier, especially at night.
    - ➤ Lubricate the anterior nasal opening with a small amount of Vaseline.
    - ➤ Avoid picking or intense blowing of the nose.
11. If bleeding reoccurs, nasal packing or cautery may be necessary.
12. For frequent nosebleeds, call for an appointment with a health care provider to evaluate the cause.

THROAT AND MOUTH ASSESSMENT

WHAT IS THE MAIN PROBLEM OR CONCERN?

How severe is it (on a scale from 0 to 5)?   When did it begin?   How is the patient responding?   Is the patient alone?

■ BLEEDING

Is the patient able to breathe, swallow, and speak?
What is the estimated amount of bleeding?
Is there drooling?

■ PAIN

Where is the exact location of the pain?
Describe the severity (on a scale from 0 to 5) and the characteristics of the
   pain (sharp, dull, or throbbing).
Are there any factors that aggravate or relieve the pain?

■ ACCOMPANYING SIGNS AND SYMPTOMS

Is there throat or mouth color changes?
Are there lesions?
Is there exudate on tonsils?
Is there fever?
Is there an earache?
Is there nasal congestion or cough?
Are there body aches?
Is a rash present?

■ HISTORY EXPOSURES

Has there been an exposure to strep throat, scarlet fever, or mononucleosis?
Has there been an exposure to flu?
Has there been an exposure to environmental irritants (smoke)?

■ HISTORY

Has there been recent trauma?
Has there been foreign body or swallowed object(s)?
Is the patient taking any prescribed or over-the-counter medications?

POSSIBLE MEDICAL PROBLEMS

Dental abscess	Mononucleosis	Thrush
Epiglottiditis	Peritonsillar abscess	Tonsillitis
Gingivitis	Scarlet fever	Tumors
Glossitis	Strep throat	Viral syndrome

TRIAGE GUIDELINES

▶ Call 911, Paramedics, or ER if:	▶ Make same-day appointment if:	▶ Call back for appointment if:
• Respiratory difficulty occurs • Tightness of throat with hives or rash develops • Inability to swallow persists • Severe mouth or throat injury occurs	• Severe sore throat persists without relief from home care measures • Sore throat develops with exudate on tonsils • High fever or earache persists • Patient is exposed to strep throat	• Signs or symptoms do not improve with home care instructions • Mouth sores or sore throat persists for >2 to 3 wk

⬢ PRECAUTIONS

- Dislodged teeth may be able to be replaced, if expedient. For example, less than 1 to 1¹/₂ hours after dislodging, bring tooth (or teeth) in container with milk, or hold in mouth, if careful not to swallow. Take to emergency room or emergency dentist.
- A direct blow to the neck may cause a fractured larynx, which may result in massive swelling and a constriction of the trachea (windpipe).
- If the patient has an extremely sore throat without the ability to swallow (drooling is present), epiglottiditis should be suspected. The individual is acutely ill and will often sit up with the mouth open and chin thrusted forward. In this case, *do not* ask the patient (or parent) to look at the throat! This may cause fatal airway obstruction. If respiratory distress occurs, send paramedics or call 911; otherwise, send directly to emergency room.

EPIGLOTTIDITIS IS MORE COMMON IN A CHILD THAN AN ADULT

- If the patient does not have the signs and symptoms of epiglottiditis (inability to swallow, drooling), look at the throat. When asking the patient to look at the throat:
  - ➤ Open mouth wide.
  - ➤ Flatten tongue, keeping tongue inside mouth.
  - ➤ Yawn.
  - ➤ Look at the throat with mirror and bright light or flashlight.

🏠 HOME CARE INSTRUCTIONS

For sore throat of recent onset without other significant signs and symptoms:

1. Gargle with ¹/₂ tsp of table salt in a glass of warm water, four to six times each day.
2. Eat or drink cold or hot foods and fluids (Popsicles, shakes, tea, broth).
3. Child–Make ice cubes with the child's favorite Kool-Aid; put in blender, or crush to make "icy."
4. Use vaporizer to sooth mucous membranes.
5. Suggest over-the-counter analgesic medications (check with health care provider).
6. If sore throat persists or if earache, high fever, or other significant signs or symptoms develop, call health care provider for an appointment.
7. Avoid environmental irritants (smoking).

For mouth sores:

1. Eat bland, cold foods and fluids.
2. Rinse mouth with warm saline solution.
3. Suggest over-the-counter analgesic medications (check with health care provider).
4. If signs or symptoms are not resolved in 2 weeks, call health care provider for an appointment.

For facial trauma:

1. Apply ice packs for swelling.
2. Suggest over-the-counter analgesic medications (check with health care

DIABETES AND BLOOD SUGAR ASSESSMENT

WHAT IS THE MAIN PROBLEM OR CONCERN?

How severe is it (on a scale from 0 to 5)?　When did it begin?　Was its onset rapid or gradual?　How is the patient responding?　Is the patient alone?

■ PHYSICAL CHARACTERISTICS

What is the condition of the skin (cool and moist or warm and dry)?

Is the pulse bounding or weak?

Is there anxiety, confusion, irritability, tremors, or personality change?

Is there faintness or headache?

Is there impaired vision?

Is there abdominal pain?

Is there nausea or vomiting?

Has there been a change in breathing pattern, or is there acetone odor to the breath?

Is there excessive thirst and appetite?

Is there excessive urination?

Are the physical characteristics mild, moderate, or severe?

Are the physical signs and symptoms stable or worsening?

■ CURRENT STATUS AND HISTORY

What is the usual daily dose of insulin? Of hypoglycemic agent?

What was the time of the last intake (insulin or oral agent)?

How does the patient measure blood sugar?

What is the current blood sugar?

What has been the pattern of control?

What was the dietary intake today?

Has there been any change in overall health status?

Has there been any change in stress or activity level?

If the patient is a woman, when was the last menstrual period?

Has there been any disease-related complications?

When did the patient last see a health care provider?

Is the patient taking prescribed or over-the-counter medications?

POSSIBLE MEDICAL PROBLEMS

Insulin shock–hypoglycemia
Too much insulin or too little food

Diabetic ketoacidosis–hyperglycemia
Not enough insulin or too much food

TRIAGE GUIDELINES

▶ Call 911, Paramedics, or ER if:	▶ Make same-day appointment if:	▶ Call back for appointment if:
• Patient is unconscious or having seizures • Blood sugar is <60 or >300 with other significant signs and symptoms • Significant signs and symptoms are present (unknown blood sugar)	• Patient is having difficulty controlling blood sugar but is in no immediate danger • Blood sugar is <60 or more >300 without other significant signs or symptoms • Mild signs and symptoms are present	• Patient experiences a change in blood sugar status • Patient develops a negative change in health status

- Signs and symptoms of hypoglycemia:
  - ➤ Sudden onset
  - ➤ Excessive sweating; cool, moist skin
  - ➤ Faintness
  - ➤ Headache
  - ➤ Pounding heart, bounding pulse
  - ➤ Anxiety, irritability
  - ➤ Confusion, personality change, slurred speech
  - ➤ Tingling of lips, tremors
  - ➤ Impaired vision
  - ➤ Headache, weakness, and faintness may occur with both hypoglycemia and hyperglycemia

⬢ PRECAUTIONS

- Hypoglycemia may progress *rapidly* to seizures or coma and death.

GIVE SOURCE OF SUGAR IMMEDIATELY
TAKE PATIENT TO THE EMERGENCY ROOM

- If individual is unable to take sugar because of nausea or vomiting, try 1 teaspoon of corn syrup or pancake syrup under the tongue. When the patient is able to drink, offer 6 ounces of Kool Aid, Coke, or other sugared drink or six gumdrops or other candy.

- If individual is not feeling better in 10 to 15 minutes, give more sugar. If possible, recheck blood sugar with home glucose meter in 15 minutes and repeat in another 15 minutes.
- Increased activity may decrease blood glucose.
- Signs and symptoms of hyperglycemia:
  - ➤ Gradual onset
  - ➤ Dry, warm skin; flushing
  - ➤ Weak pulse
  - ➤ Abdominal pain
  - ➤ Nausea and vomiting
  - ➤ Rapid deep breathing with acetone odor
  - ➤ Thirst and increased urination

⬢ PRECAUTIONS

- Hyperglycemia may progress to coma and death.
- Infection, pregnancy, or severe anxiety may elevate blood glucose.

NEEDS INSULIN
TAKE PATIENT TO THE EMERGENCY ROOM
OR MAKE SAME-DAY APPOINTMENT FOR MILD SIGNS OR SYMPTOMS

Diabetes and
blood sugar

MALE GENITOURINARY ASSESSMENT

WHAT IS THE MAIN PROBLEM OR CONCERN?

How severe is it (on a scale from 0 to 5)?   When did it begin?   How is the patient responding?

■ PENILE

Describe the pain or discomfort, if any.
Is there a discharge? If so, what is the color and amount. Is there odor?
Is there swelling?
Is there a rash or itching?
Are there lesions or blisters?
Is there a blue or gray discoloration?

■ TESTICLE

Describe the pain or discomfort, if any.
Is there swelling or lumps?
Is there a rash or itching?
Are there lesions or blisters?
Is there a blue or gray discoloration?

■ URINARY SYMPTOMS

Is there pain with urination?
Is there an urgency or a frequency of urination?
Are there problems starting the stream of urine?
Does the patient believe that there is retention of urine?
Is there blood in the urine?
Is there abdominal, lower back, or flank pain?
Is there fever?

■ HISTORY

Has there been recent trauma?
Is there possible exposure to sexually transmitted disease?
Are there chronic health conditions? Has there been recent surgery, diagnostic procedure, or hospitalization?
What medications, prescribed and over-the-counter, is the patient taking?

POSSIBLE MEDICAL PROBLEMS	
Epididymitis	Tinea cruris (jock itch)
Prostatitis	*Pediatric:*
Sexually transmitted infections	Sexual abuse
Testicular torsion	

TRIAGE GUIDELINES

▶ Call 911, Paramedics, or ER if:	▶ Make same-day appointment if:	▶ Call back for appointment if:
• Patient has experienced a severe injury • Severe groin pain or edema persists, especially if there is a sudden onset or a sudden decrease of pain • Blue or gray discoloration develops • Patient is unable to void and medical office is closed	• Moderate pain, dysuria, discharge, rash, or itching develops • There is possible exposure to a sexually transmitted disease • Patient is unable to void bladder and has mild discomfort	• Signs or symptoms do not improve with home care instructions • Other significant signs or symptoms develop

⬤ PRECAUTIONS

- In cases of testicular torsion, immediate surgery may be necessary.
- If severe testicular pain or swelling develops, take nothing by mouth.
- Avoid sexual activities before medical evaluation.

Pediatric considerations:

- Consider sexual abuse.
- For male newborn, blood-tinged urine may occur and should subside within 1 day.

⌂ HOME CARE INSTRUCTIONS *(for mild rash and itching irritation without exposure to a sexually transmitted disease)*

1. Apply Caldesene or another brand of baby powder to affected area after daily bath or shower.
2. Wear white supportive cotton underwear day and night and loose, baggy clothing.
3. Avoid activities that may cause excessive perspiration.
4. If signs or symptoms persist, call back for appointment.

FEMALE GENITOURINARY ASSESSMENT

WHAT IS THE MAIN PROBLEM OR CONCERN?

How severe is it (on a scale from 0 to 5)?   When did it begin?   How is the patient responding?

■ URINARY SYMPTOMS

Is there an urgency or a frequency of urination? Is there dysuria?
What are the characteristics of the urine (hematuria, cloudiness, or unusual odor)?

■ ACCOMPANYING SIGNS AND SYMPTOMS

Is there fever?
Is there back or flank pain?
Is there pain or pressure in the lower abdomen or pelvic area?

■ EXTERNAL GENITAL SIGNS AND SYMPTOMS

Is there itching or burning?
Is there a discharge? If so, describe the color and characteristics.
Is there pain, bleeding, lesions, or lacerations?

■ HISTORY

Is there a history of trauma or possible abuse?
Has there been exposure to a sexually transmitted disease?
Is there a history of urinary tract infections?
What method of birth control is the patient using?
Has there been use of antibiotics within the past 6 weeks?
What medications, prescribed and over-the-counter, is the patient taking?

POSSIBLE MEDICAL PROBLEMS

Menstrual flow after birth	Straddle injury	*Pregnancy complications:*	*Pediatric:*
Pyelonephritis	Urinary tract infection	Premature labor	Sexual abuse
Sexually transmitted disease	Vaginitis		

TRIAGE GUIDELINES

▶ Call 911, Paramedics, or ER if:	▶ Make same-day appointment if:	▶ Call back for appointment if:
• Rape or trauma has occurred *Pediatric considerations:* • Child abuse is suspected (refer to the state and county guidelines for reporting child abuse) Follow up if child is not checked in at ER	• Moderate to severe burning on urination persists • Urination is frequent and urgent • Moderate to severe vaginal signs and symptoms persist • There has been exposure to sexually transmitted diseases	• Vaginal or urinary signs or symptoms do not improve with home care instructions • Other significant signs or symptoms develop • Possible exposure to a sexually transmitted disease has occurred

⬟ PRECAUTIONS

- Avoid putting anything (douching, creams, or foams) in the vagina before medical assessment. Avoid intercourse.

Pre-ER Instructions

➤ In the case of rape, avoid bathing or changing clothes.

➤ In the case of rape, recommend that a family member or friend drive the patient to an emergency room.

🏠 HOME CARE INSTRUCTIONS

For mild vaginal signs and symptoms with no exposure to sexually transmitted disease:

1. Soak in warm or cool bath for 20 minutes.
2. Wear loose cotton underwear and clothing.
3. Pour warm water over genitals while voiding to decrease discomfort, or urinate in a warm bath.
4. If vaginal itching and "cheesy" white discharge are present, the patient may have a vaginal yeast infection. Advise that there are over-the-counter medications for treatment. Recommend that the patient check with her health care provider.

For mild urinary symptoms:

1. Drink 8 to 10 glasses of fluid a day, including cranberry juice. Avoid coffee, tea, alcohol, and caffeinated drinks; they may cause irritation to the bladder.
2. Avoid perfumed sprays, soaps, bath oils, and colored toilet tissue.
3. Urinate after intercourse.
4. Cleanse genitals with mild soap and warm water after intercourse. Always clean genital area from front to back.
5. Never "hold" urine; bacteria may multiply. Urinate as frequently as necessary.
6. If signs or symptoms continue or increase, call back for an appointment.

Pediatric considerations:

- For female newborn, reassure parent that if the child is having no other signs or symptoms, mild vaginal bleeding is normal and should subside.

GYNECOLOGIC ASSESSMENT

WHAT IS THE MAIN PROBLEM OR CONCERN?

How severe is it (on a scale from 0 to 5)?　When did it begin?　How is the patient responding?

■ BLEEDING

What is the amount of the bleeding? How many pads or tampons were changed today?

Did the bleeding begin after coitus or after a bowel movement?

Is there passage of clots or tissue? If so, what is the size of the clot or tissue?

When was the last normal menstrual period? When was the period before that?

■ PAIN

What is the exact location of the pain?

Describe the characteristics and severity (on a scale from 0 to 5) of the pain or discomfort. Is the pain diffuse or localized? Constant or intermittent? Sharp or dull? Is the pain a cramp, or does it throb?

Are there areas that are tender to the touch?

Are there any factors that aggravate or relieve the symptoms?

■ URINARY SIGNS AND SYMPTOMS

Is there an urgency or a frequency of urination? Is there dysuria?

What are the characteristics of the urine (hematuria, cloudiness, or an unusual odor)?

Is there back or flank pain?

Is there pain or pressure in the abdominal or pelvic areas?

■ VAGINAL SIGNS AND SYMPTOMS

Is there a discharge? If so, describe the color, amount, and characteristics.

Is there itching or burning?

Is there odor?

Are there lesions or lacerations?

■ ACCOMPANYING SIGNS AND SYMPTOMS

Is there a fever?

Is there a feeling of lightheadedness or dizziness?

■ HISTORY

Is there a history of trauma?

Is there possible exposure to sexually transmitted disease?

What method of birth control is the patient using?

Are there chronic health conditions, such as pelvic inflammatory disease or endometriosis?

Has there been recent pelvic surgery, diagnostic procedure, or hospitalization?

When was the date of the last gynecologic examination and Pap smear? What were the results of the examination?

What medications, prescribed and over-the-counter, is the patient taking?

POSSIBLE MEDICAL PROBLEMS

Amenorrhea	Dysmenorrhea	Pregnancy–uterine or ectopic	Gonorrhea	*Vaginitis:*
Cancer of the cervix, uterus, or ovaries	Endometriosis or Endometritis	Salpingitis	Herpes	Atrophy
	Fibroids	Torsion of adnexal mass	Human immunodeficiency virus	Bacterial vaginosis
Corpus luteum cyst	Menorrhagia	*Sexually transmitted diseases:*	Hepatitis B	Candida (Monilia or yeast)
Dysfunctional bleeding	Pelvic inflammatory disease	Chlamydia	Syphilis	Trichomoniasis

TRIAGE GUIDELINES

▶ Call 911, Paramedics, or ER if:	▶ Make same-day appointment if:	▶ Call back for appointment if:
• Severe vaginal bleeding develops (soaking one or more full-sized maxi-pads every 30 minutes for ≥2 hr), especially with weakness or dizziness • Pregnant, any bloody flow develops; if >20 weeks pregnant, go to L&D • Rape or trauma has occurred • Severe pelvic pain persists with signs and symptoms of shock (significant weakness, dizziness, or sweating)	• Unexplained out-of-cycle vaginal bleeding begins • Painful urination persists • Moderate to severe vaginal signs and symptoms continue • Exposure to sexually transmitted disease is possible • Moderate pelvic pain exists	• Vaginal bleeding continues over a 10-day period • Midcycle pelvic pain continues >2 days or increases with or without other significant signs and symptoms

⬢ PRECAUTIONS

- Pregnancy should be a consideration for all women of childbearing years, even those individuals who had a bilateral tubal ligation.
- Consider possible ruptured ectopic pregnancy, a condition that may be life threatening.
- A patient with an ectopic pregnancy may report nausea and vomiting and shoulder, upper chest, or back pain.
- Severe right or left lower-quadrant pain may indicate ovarian cysts or appendicitis. Rupture may cause peritonitis.
- Avoid douches, creams, foams, or intercourse until medical evaluation.
- If patient is taking birth control pills, breakthrough bleeding is common in the first 3 months. If pills are taken late or missed, vaginal bleeding or spotting is common.
- If patient is taking Depo-Provera injections or Norplant for birth control, irregular vaginal spotting or light bleeding is common.
- Out-of-cycle bleeding or spotting may indicate a sexually transmitted disease, an undiagnosed pregnancy, a hormonal imbalance, a cervical polyp, or uterine or cervical cancer.
- Use menstrual pads only, no tampons.

Pre-ER Instructions

➤ If tissue is passed, the patient should be instructed to save the tissue and take it to the emergency room.

➤ If there is heavy bleeding, recommend that a family member or friend drive the patient to the emergency room. The patient should lie down in the back seat of the car and elevate feet.

🏠 HOME CARE INSTRUCTIONS

For heavy menses:

1. Rest with feet up.
2. Encourage patient to increase liquid intake.
3. Bleeding should begin to decrease within 1 to 2 hours.

For mild midcycle pelvic pain:

1. Right or left lower-quadrant midcycle pain may indicate ovulation. Without other significant signs and symptoms, this pain should be gone in 1 to 2 days.
2. Patient may use a heating pad on lower abdominal area.
3. Encourage an over-the-counter analgesic. Patient should check with her health care provider.
4. If pain persists or if other signs and symptoms develop, encourage patient to make an appointment for evaluation.
5. Hypogastric pain may indicate an urinary tract infection. Question the patient regarding painful urination, frequency, and urgency.

35

OBSTETRIC ASSESSMENT

WHAT IS THE MAIN PROBLEM OR CONCERN?

How severe is it (on a scale from 0 to 5)?   When did it begin?   When was the patient's last normal menstrual period?
How many weeks gestation or what is the estimated date of confinement?   How is the patient responding to the problem?   Is the patient alone?

■ BLEEDING

What is the amount and color of the bleeding (staining or flow)?
Did the bleeding begin after coitus or after a bowel movement?
Is there passage of clots or tissue? If so, what is the size of the clot or tissue?
Is there weakness, dizziness, or sweating?

■ PAIN, CRAMPING, AND CONTRACTIONS

What is the exact location of the pain?
Does the pain radiate to other parts of the body?
How severe is the pain (on a scale from 0 to 5)?
How frequently does the pain occur?
Are there any factors that aggravate or relieve the symptoms?
If the patient is less than 20 weeks gestational age, is there shoulder, lower back, or upper unilateral chest pain?

■ VAGINAL SIGNS AND SYMPTOMS

Is there a discharge? If so, describe the color, amount, and characteristics.
Is there odor?
Is there itching or burning?
Are there lesions or lacerations?
Is there vaginal pressure? Is fetal part or cord protruding?

■ URINARY SIGNS AND SYMPTOMS

Is there a frequency or an urgency of urination? Is there dysuria?
What are the characteristics of the urine (hematuria, cloudiness, or an unusual odor)?
Is there pain in the back or flank or in the abdominal or pelvic areas?
Is there a fever?

■ IF MORE THAN 20 WEEKS GESTATIONAL AGE

Is there headache pain? Is there epigastric pain? Is there edema of the hands or face? Are there visual disturbances? Is there dizziness?
If the patient is more than 28 weeks gestational age, has there been a change in fetal movements?

■ HISTORY

Has an intrauterine pregnancy been confirmed by a pelvic examination or sonogram?
Are there chronic health conditions? Is the patient on medication?
Is this a twin or an increased risk pregnancy?
Has there been recent trauma, diagnostic screening tests, or hospitalization?

POSSIBLE MEDICAL PROBLEMS

Sexually transmitted disease	*Less than 20 weeks LNMP:*	Hyperemesis gravidarum	*More than 20 weeks LNMP:*	Pregnancy induced hypertension
Urinary tract infection	Ectopic pregnancy	Missed abortion	Abruptio placenta	Premature rupture of membranes
Vaginal infection	(usually under 8 weeks)	Round ligament syndrome (pull)	Hemorrhage or shock	Preterm labor
	Hemorrhage or shock	Spontaneous abortion	Hyperemesis gravidarum	Round ligament syndrome
	Hydatidiform mole	Threatened abortion	Labor	Rupture of membranes
			Placenta previa	

TRIAGE GUIDELINES

▶ Call 911, Paramedics, or ER L&D if:

- Vaginal bleeding begins, similar to a menstrual period *(if tissue is passed, patient should take the tissue to the ER)*
- Regular contractions or abdominal, pelvic, or back pain is not relieved by a warm shower, relaxation, or rest on the left side
- Fetal movement is <3-4/hr after eating *(if >28 wk)*
- Watery vaginal discharge or rupture of membranes begins *(>20 wk)*
- Anything protrudes from the vagina *(assume the knee-to-chest position; do not attempt to push anything back into the vagina)*
- Severe headache, visual disturbances, or sudden edema or disorientation develops

▶ Make same-day appointment if:

- *Caution:* Do not bring a patient in active labor, actively bleeding, or in acute distress to an office or clinic setting; go to ER if <20 wk, L&D if >20 wk
- Unexplained vaginal spotting, staining, or vaginal flow *(>20 wk)* should be evaluated in L&D
- Minor vaginal spotting or staining begins *(<20 wk)* without other significant signs or symptoms
- Mild to moderate pelvic or abdominal pain develops with no relief when resting *(<20 wk)* without bleeding or other significant signs or symptoms

▶ Call back for appointment if:

- Recommend the safest alternative–bring the patient in for evaluation
- Health status changes
- Fetal movements decrease *(>28 wk)*
- Anxiety continues *(may need to be checked for fetal heart tones to reassure mother)*

■ TRIAGE CONSIDERATIONS AND INSTRUCTIONS

- Consider the severity of the signs and symptoms and the ability of the patient to drive herself. The patient may require a driver, ambulance, or paramedic transportation to the hospital.
- Signs and symptoms of shock include dizziness, nausea, or vomiting and pale, moist, cool skin.
- Consider that the patient with multiple signs and symptoms is usually more urgent.
- Signs and symptoms of an ectopic pregnancy include right or left lower-quadrant pain, upper abdominal pain, or shoulder, unilateral chest, or back pain. (May be life threatening!)
- Laying on the left side decreases pressure on the vena cava and increases oxygen supply to the fetus and maternal major organs.
- Minor vaginal staining or spotting in early pregnancy may be caused by an increased vascularity of the tissues. Staining or spotting is more common after coitus or bowel movement but may occur at other times.

More than 28 weeks pregnant (patient needs to be seen immediately):
- A decrease in fetal activity should be monitored.
- If the patient reports a green vaginal discharge, consider meconium staining and ruptured membranes.
- Edema of the face and hands may indicate pregnancy-induced hypertension. Epigastric pain, headache, visual disturbances, and disorientation may indicate impending seizure.
- Regular contractions that increase in frequency, duration, and intensity and water leakage from the vagina are signs of impending delivery.
  1. Instruct patient to lie on her left side.
  2. Avoid pushing, and practice breathing techniques when the sensation to push begins–"he-he-he-who" or panting with each contraction.
  3. If the mother feels the need to bear down or have a bowel movement, if she is experiencing heavy bloody flow, frequent contractions, bulging membranes from the vulva, or fetal head crowning, birth is imminent. Call 911 operator, physician, or a certified nurse midwife to instruct mother or caller. Do not allow mother to sit on toilet.

PERIANAL ASSESSMENT

WHAT IS THE MAIN PROBLEM OR CONCERN?

How severe is it (on a scale from 0 to 5)?   When did it begin?   How is the patient responding?

■ PERIANAL PAIN CHARACTERISTICS

Describe the pain or discomfort. Is the pain an ache or is it a burning sensation? Sharp or dull? Is the pain a cramp or does it throb?

Is the pain external or internal?

Are there factors that may aggravate or relieve the symptoms?

Is there itching?

Is there edema?

Is there bleeding? If so, what is its frequency and amount?

Are there lesions or blisters?

Is there a rash?

■ HISTORY

Are there chronic health conditions such as hemorrhoids, fissures, or polyps?

Has there been recent trauma?

Are there sexual practices that may contribute to the signs and symptoms?

Is it possible that a foreign object is embedded?

Have there been recent changes in bowel habits?

If the patient is a child, is he or she restless at night?

Is the patient taking any prescribed or over-the-counter medications?

POSSIBLE MEDICAL PROBLEMS

Constipation	Rectal tumor	*Pediatric:*
Fissures	Sexually transmitted infections	Diaper rash
Hemorrhoids	Sexual practice–related abuse	Sexual abuse
Parasitic infections (pinworms)		

TRIAGE GUIDELINES

▶ Call 911, Paramedics, or ER if:	▶ Make same-day appointment if:	▶ Call back for appointment if:
• Severe perianal injury, rape, or abscess occurs • Profuse or uncontrolled bleeding develops • Foreign object is embedded	• Moderate to severe pain persists • Itching, rash, or edema persists • Exposure to a sexually transmitted disease is possible	• Perianal signs or symptoms do not improve with home care instructions • Other significant signs or symptoms develop

🏠 HOME CARE INSTRUCTIONS

For mild rash and itching with no exposure to a sexually transmitted disease:

1. Patient should bathe or shower daily.
2. Patient should dry completely after bathing and blow dry area with dryer on cool setting. Instruct patient to apply Caldesene or another brand of baby powder.
3. Patient should wear clean white, cotton underwear and loose baggy clothing.
4. If signs and symptoms (itching, rash, edema, pain, bleeding, lesions, blisters) persist, call a health care provider for an appointment.
5. If there is a history of hemorrhoids and if the patient believes the signs and symptoms are related:
   ➤ Soak in warm bathtub for 20 to 30 minutes two to three times each day.
   ➤ Advise the patient of several over-the-counter medications for the relief of signs and symptoms (patient should check with his or her health care provider).
   ➤ Advise the patient to avoid constipation by (1) maintaining adequate fluid intake, (2) avoiding white flour products, and (3) increasing fresh fruits and vegetables, as well as whole grain foods.
6. If the patient (or parent) can see pinworms (pinworms are active at night) or if there is rectal itching and restlessness, encourage the patient to call a health care provider for recommendation of treatment.

For diarrhea:

1. See Gastrointestinal assessment and triage guidelines (pp. 6-7)

Pediatric instructions for mild to moderate diaper rash:

- Frequently change diapers.
- Use plain water to clean diaper area after changing; do not use diaper wipes.
- Allow infant to go without a diaper at least 1 hour after each diaper change.
- Maintain a loose diaper.
- Use over-the-counter creams or ointments at bedtime (check with a health care provider).
- For the prevention of diaper rash, use Caldesene or another brand of baby powder.
- See a health care provider if the rash is not improved in 24 hours or if the rash becomes worse. Always see a health care provider for severe diaper rash with bleeding.
- If diarrhea is the cause of the diaper rash, diarrhea must be treated. If infant or child has an oral yeast infection (thrush), rash needs to be treated with medication. (Check with a health care provider.)

PSYCHOSOCIAL ASSESSMENT

WHAT IS THE MAIN PROBLEM OR CONCERN?

When did it begin?   How severe is it (on a scale from 0 to 5)?   How are the signs and symptoms affecting daily functioning?

■ LETHAL RISK QUESTIONS

Ask the following questions to determine if there is a risk of suicide

Are you alone? *(Obtain location and verify address)*

Have you had thoughts about ending your life? *(If yes)* Have you thought about how you would do it?

Ask the following questions to determine if suicide is currently a serious risk

Do you have that nearby? *(Attempt to have the patient put the item[s] away)*

How much time do we have?

Ask the following questions to attempt to get the caller to agree to a verbal contract with you

Will you promise me that you will be okay until I can arrange for a counselor to speak with you (over telephone or in office)?

Will you promise me that you will not harm yourself without first calling back here?

■ CURRENT STATUS: PHYSICAL SIGNS AND SYMPTOMS

Have you heard sounds or seen things that others do not hear or see?

Is there use of drugs or alcohol? If yes, is the patient under the influence at this time? What substance is the patient using? When was the substance last used and what amount?

Have there been palpitations, chest pain, shortness of breath, or shakiness or dizziness?

Is there vomiting, diarrhea, or abdominal pain?

How is the individual's appetite?

Has there been a recent weight loss?

What is the patient's current weight and height?

Describe the individual's sleeping pattern.

What successful coping mechanism has the patient previously used?

Can the patient identify supportive people?

■ HISTORY

Is there a history of counseling? Current or past?

Is there a social support system (family, friends, neighbors, church)?

Is there a history of anxiety attacks or panic disorders?

Is there a history of previous suicide attempts?

Is there a terminal or chronic disease?

If a woman:

Did the patient recently give birth?

If a child:

Has there been any behavioral changes recently?

Has there been a recent change or loss in the household, school, or close relationship (marital separation, new family member)?

Is there a history of abuse or molestation?

Is there a history of depression or other psychologic problems?

Is there a history of trauma?

Is there an exposure to drugs, alcohol, or environmental substances? If yes, what substance is the patient using or been exposed to? When was the substance last used and what amount?

POSSIBLE PSYCHOSOCIAL PROBLEMS

Affective disorder	Attention deficit disorder	Developmental delays	Panic reactions	Postpartum depression psychosis
Alcoholic hallucinosis	Chemical dependency	Manic episodes	Paranoid personality disorders	Posttraumatic stress disorder
Anorexia or bulimia	Depression (with or without	Obsessive compulsive disorder	Personality disorders	Schizophrenia
Anxiety	suicide attempts or thoughts)	Organic brain syndrome	Phobias	Seasonal affective disorder

TRIAGE GUIDELINES

► Call 911, Paramedics, or ER if:	► Make same-day appointment if:	► Call back for appointment if:
• Patient has a weapon or plans to harm self or another 　› Obtain correct address 　› Stay on the telephone with the caller until the police arrive 　› If no address is given, the call may be traced • Patient is suicidal or is experiencing auditory or visual hallucinations • Severe and crippling anxiety develops • Patient is experiencing panic or terror and is unable to be calmed • Patient is under the influence of drugs and alcohol • Significant physical sign and symptoms are present	• Severe insomnia or depression develops • Life crisis has occurred • Lose of appetite has caused a significant weight loss • Severe anxiety develops without relief from a support system or if no support system is available • Moderate physical signs and symptoms are present	• Negative change occurs in mental, emotional, or physical status

⬤ PRECAUTIONS

- Suicide thoughts, plans, and items readily available (weapon, pills) indicate the individual is at risk of following through with the plan. Write a note to a co-worker to call 911 or the police while you stay on the telephone with the patient after verifying address.
- If the patient does not have a plan, conclude the call with a verbal contract, "I want you to promise you will not harm yourself without first calling here. Will you please promise me that?" Arrange for the patient to speak with a mental health provider or suicide hotline as soon as possible.
- Show the caller that you care and wish to understand more about the patient's feelings.
- Allow the patient to ventilate feelings, past losses, and current life challenges.
- Provide crisis "hot" or "warm" lines to the caller with psychosocial problems.
- Do not offer advice or false hopes to the patient.
- Always invite and encourage the individual to call back if needed.
- Make a follow-up call the next day, if possible.

For the individual without significant physical signs and symptoms but in need of ventilation, coping mechanisms, a support system and resources, refer to a mental health professional. Current lists of community support groups, battered women's shelter referral lines, and other crises groups should be available to the triage nurse.

PEDIATRIC ILLNESS
TRIAGE GUIDELINES

▶ **Call 911, Paramedics, or ER if:**

- Child develops respiratory distress
- Uncontrolled high fever with rigid stiff neck
- Seizure occurs without fever
- Medical office is closed or if the parent is unable to obtain a same-day appointment and the child is acutely ill
- Severe lethargy with poor eye contact persists

▶ **Make same-day appointment if:**

- Fever is not controlled by cooling measures or is >103° F
- *Any* fever is present in an infant <2 mo of age
- Fever >100.5° F persists >3 days
- Lethargy with poor eye contact persists
- Febrile seizure develops
- Severe nasal congestion persists without improvement with home care measures
- Severe cough and chest congestion with green sputum develops
- Wheezing persists without improvement with health provider's prescription
- Severe sore throat continues with or without strep exposure
- Uncontrolled vomiting (>2 hr) or diarrhea (>4 hr) continues without improvement with home care measures
- Child is listless and refuses foods or fluids for >4 hr
- Child is pulling or tugging at ear or complaining of earache
- Suspicious rash develops (refer to Common Childhood Rashes, p. 46)
- Parent requests that child be seen

▶ **Call back for appointment if:**

- Child does not improve with home care measures
- Additional signs or symptoms develop
- Child is not "well" within a reasonable length of time or continues with frequent illnesses
- Parental anxiety exists

⬢ PRECAUTIONS

- Parents may be anxious and overreact to their child's condition; however, they may also have a "sixth sense." Remember, the parent is the child's only advocate. A parent with anxiety that appears out of proportion to the child's described condition may be unable to verbalize the child's true condition or "know" their child is seriously ill.

BE CAUTIOUS
ADVISE PARENT TO BRING THE CHILD TO A HEALTH CARE PROVIDER

🏠 HOME CARE INSTRUCTIONS

Home care instructions should be given to the parents of an infant or a child who has a mild illness of recent onset.or to the parents for use before the child can be evaluated by a health care provider. (For gastrointestinal, respiratory, or problems with other systems, please see appropriate assessment.)

1. Cooling measures: Fever higher than 102.5° F
   A. Tylenol–dose for weight and age (check with health care provider).
   B. If child is trembling with chills
      1. Wrap warm blanket around the child's lower legs and feet only.
      2. Apply lukewarm water to the child's head.
   C. When child is not trembling
      1. Place child in lukewarm bath for 30 minutes with head and hair thoroughly wet.
      2. If child is not vomiting, offer liquids (Kool Aid, Popsicle, water) to drink while in warm bath.
      3. After bath, dress child in light clothing.
      4. Involve child in quiet activities such as reading or watching television.
      5. Recheck temperature 15 minutes after bathing. Temperature should decrease 1° to 2° F. If fever has not decreased, repeat warm bath and encourage additional fluids.
      6. If fever still has not decreased, child should be seen by a health care provider the same day.
2. Restful activities: Ill children should be provided with quiet activities in a quiet environment. Encourage reading, coloring, board games, or watching television with napping. If signs and symptoms do not improve within 3 days or if other signs and symptoms develop, the child should be seen by a health care provider.

CHILD ABUSE AND NEGLECT ASSESSMENT

■ DESCRIPTION OF ALLEGED ABUSE AND NEGLECT

What is the extent of injury to the child?

Describe the condition and behavior of the child at this time.

How does the caller know of the alleged abuse or neglect?

What is the date and location of the alleged abuse or neglect?

Where is the child now?

Is the child now in a safe environment?

Are there other children in the family?

What is the location of the alleged abuser now?

What is the name of the caller and his or her relationship to the family?

What is the telephone number and address of the caller? Of the child? Of the alleged abuser?

If an individual is abusing a child, there is a high probability that more than one child or person is being abused by that individual. If there is physical child abuse, there may also be spousal abuse.

Substance abuse and major family stresses may be involved. Also, there may be transient persons in the home.

Types of child abuse:

- Physical
- Sexual
- Verbal
- Emotional
- Neglect

TRIAGE GUIDELINES

▶ Call 911, Police, Child Abuse Authorities, or ER if:	▶ Make same-day appointment if:	▶ Call back for appointment if:
• Child is in the process of being abused or neglected at the time of the call	• Abuse is suspected, but no evidence exists, and child has no physical signs or symptoms; parent needs to discuss situation with a health care provider	• Child must be seen for evaluation
Obtain correct address		
Follow the mandated laws of the state for reporting alleged abuse or neglect		

• Child abuse registry hotlines
  • County public health department
  • Social service		

Discuss immediate options to obtain safe environment for child		

■ DESCRIPTION OF ALLEGED ABUSE

Has anyone ever hurt or frightened you? Describe the incident.

What was the extent of the injury?

How would you describe your condition at this time?

Was this reported to the police or another agency?

Do you have family, friends, or neighbors who can help you?

When was the last time this happened?

Are you now in a safe environment?

Are you alone?

Where is the abuser now?

Make adult aware of their own resources (family, friends, neighbors)

Encourage individual to call someone who has been supportive to them in the past.

Types of adult abuse:
- Physical
- Sexual
- Verbal
- Emotional
- Neglect (if ill, disabled, or elderly)

Have a list of the battered adult shelter hotline, "warm" lines, and family crises lines.

Be aware that if an adult is abusing one person in the household, there is a high probability that more than one person is being abused. If there is spousal abuse, there also may be child abuse. Often these families have chronic problems with unemployment, alcoholism, and drug abuse. Also, there may be transient persons in and out of the home.

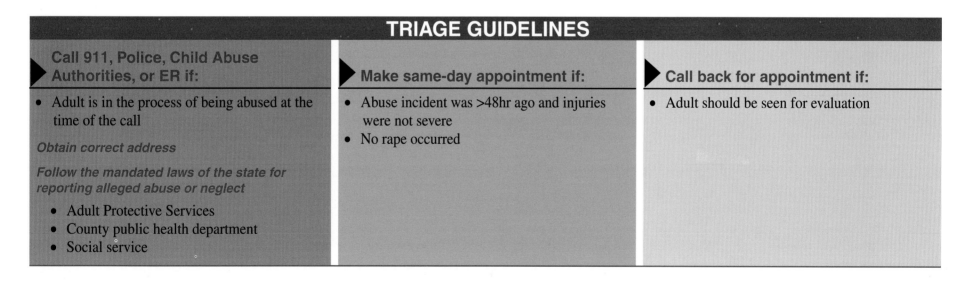

TRIAGE GUIDELINES

▶ Call 911, Police, Child Abuse Authorities, or ER if:	▶ Make same-day appointment if:	▶ Call back for appointment if:

• Adult is in the process of being abused at the time of the call
 	
Obtain correct address
 	
Follow the mandated laws of the state for reporting alleged abuse or neglect
  • Adult Protective Services
  • County public health department
  • Social service
	• Abuse incident was >48hr ago and injuries were not severe
	• No rape occurred
		• Adult should be seen for evaluation

ASSESSMENT OF COMMON CHILDHOOD RASHES

Rash	Fever	Itching	Elevation	Color	Location	Duration	Other symptoms
Prickly heat	No	Sometimes	Slightly raised dots	White or red dots; surrounding skin may be red	Trunk, neck, skin on arms and legs	Until controlled	
Diaper rash	No	No	Only if infected	Red	Under diaper	Until controlled	
Impetigo	Some-times	Occasionally	Crusts on sores	Golden crusts on red sores	Arms, legs, face first; then most of body	Until controlled	
Ringworm	No	Occasionally	Slightly raised rings	Red	Anywhere, including scalp and nails	Until controlled	Flaking or scaling
Hives	No	Intense	Raised with flat tops	Pale raised lesions surrounded by red	Anywhere	Minutes to days	
Poison ivy	No	Intense	Blisters are elevated	Red	Exposed areas	7-14 days	Oozing; some swelling
Eczema	No	Moderate to intense	Occasional blisters when infected	Red	Elbows, wrists, knees, cheeks	Until controlled	Moist; oozing
Acne	No	No	Pimples, cysts	Red	Face, back, chest	Until controlled	Blackheads
Athlete's foot	No	Mild to intense	No	Colorless to red	Between toes	Until controlled	Cracks; scaling; oozing blisters
Scabies	No	Intense	Slight	Red crusting	Arms, legs, trunk; Infant: head, neck, hands, feet	Until controlled	
Cradle cap and dandruff	No	Occasionally	Some crusting	White to yellow to red	Scalp, eyebrows, behind ears, groin	Until controlled	Fine, oily scales
Chicken pox	Yes	Intense during pustular stage	Flat, then raised, then blisters, then crusts	Red	May start anywhere; most prominent on trunk and face	4-10 days	Lesions progress from flat to blisters, then become crusted
Measles	Yes	None to mild	Flat	Pink, then red	First face, then chest and abdomen, then arms and legs	4-7 days	Preceded by fever, cough, red eyes
German measles (Rubella)	Yes	No	Flat or slightly raised	Red	First face, then trunk, then extremities	2-4 days	Swollen glands behind ears; occasional joint pains in older children
Roseola	Yes	No	Flat, occasionally with a few bumps	Pink	First trunk, then arms and neck; very little on face and legs	1-2 days	High fever for 3 days that disappears with rash
Scarlet fever	Yes	No	Flat; feels like sandpaper	Red	First face, then elbows; spreads rapidly to entire body in 24 hours	5-7 days	Sore throat; skin peeling afterward, especially palms
Fifth disease	No	No	Flat; lacy appearance	Red	First face, then arms and legs, then rest of body	3-7 days	"Slapped-cheek" appearance; rash comes and goes

Pentell, Fries, Vickery: *Taking care of your child*, ed 3 (table H), ©1990 by Addison-Wesley Publishing Co,. Inc. Reprinted by permission.